Why
Children
Sit Still?

Why Don't Children Sit Still?

A Parent's Guide to Healthy Movement and Play in Child Development

Evelien van Dort

Floris Books

Translated by Barbara Mees

First published in Dutch as *Bewegen – Eerst je lijf in,
dan de wereld in* by Uitgeverij Christofoor in 2016
First published in English by Floris Books in 2018
© 2016 Uitgeverij Christofoor, Zeist
English version © 2018 Floris Books

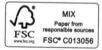

 Also available as an eBook

British Library CIP data available
ISBN 978-178250-514-3
Printed in Great Britain
by TJ International

CONTENTS

PART 3: MOVEMENT AND LEARNING

Introduction

I'm on my way to a house call. In the middle of the road in front of me, a little boy is riding his bike behind his father. He races past his father and pedals as if his life depends on it. A car stops to let him pass. His father thanks the driver by giving him a thumbs up, as the boy carefully steers around the car. I catch myself being critical. Can a small child pedal, steer and be aware of traffic all at the same time? Safe on the pavement now, our young hero jumps from his bike and triumphantly waits for his father, eyes shining and cheeks rosy.

To answer my question above about the capabilities of the little boy, I first need to introduce two concepts: *sensorimotor development* and *sensorimotor coupling*. Children move from the moment they arrive in the world. Through movement and the use of their senses, they experience and learn about themselves and the world around them. This is called *sensorimotor development*, which can only be achieved through *sensorimotor coupling* – the integration of sensory observation and bodily movement. Put another way, it's the body's physical reaction to information obtained through the senses. Our central nervous system (the brain and spinal cord) combines all of these complex processes. In the case of our little boy, he saw a car approaching so braked and steered around it. The sensory input produced a motor output.

However, although it looks like he can cycle well – he steers and pedals without any problems – there's a good chance that should he see something interesting on the left, he'll be distracted, steer to the left and leave the path, putting him in danger. His sense of balance, connected to the movement of his head and his hands on the handlebars, can't yet be used separately so he may fall. If a car approaches him, he will have to determine when to brake or steer away. Judging the speed of a car is a difficult motor process, which includes bodily movement and complex processing of sensory information. I believe my anxiety at the situation was justified.

Sensorimotor coupling is the basis for all learning. Some may think this is a well-kept secret, but the truth is that the relationship between movement and cognitive learning has been known for quite some time. The ancient Greeks walked while learning poetry by heart, a practice reflected in recent brain research showing that primary school children perform better if they move while learning. Of course, the world of education has many different opinions regarding the 'best' way to learn, and as a result has created as many educational systems. One of these is the Steiner-Waldorf approach, based on the theories of anthroposophy, which I will refer to throughout this book. Moving while learning is an integral part of the Waldorf approach to learning.

Movement in combination with experience will give young children, and even adolescents, an invaluable physical base. But sensorimotor development is too often forgotten. In this book I will explain how it forms the basis for healthy child development in all areas. For example, when looking for answers to concerns relating to other areas of a child's physical and socio-emotional progression, it can often help to look closely at their sensorimotor development.

Child development can be compared to the process of ripening – it takes time. Too often we see this ripening process put under pressure, either from over-generalised development targets or through social influence, for example: 'All the kids in my class have swimming lessons' or 'Doesn't your child cycle without training wheels yet?' We live in a fast-paced world and our children have to move with it, but they need time to rest and process daily life. It can be difficult to practise, but exertion should always be followed by relaxation. First and foremost, every child is unique and therefore develops in their own unique way. Learning to look at the way a specific child moves helps us to offer the kinds of movement that suit them best, for example playing a particular sport or musical instrument.

I have been practising children's physiotherapy for the past thirty years, during which time I have been asked many different questions on the relationship between sensorimotor skills and child development: 'My seven-year-old has poor handwriting, would typing on a computer be a good solution?' Or: 'My ten-and-a-half-year-old has an injury and has not been able to play football for six months, should she try another sport?' My starting point is always to look at each child individually and holistically.

In this book, I combine the experiences gained in my practice with theories and insights from mainstream, anthroposophical and holistic medicine. There are tips and facts to help parents and educators, as well as frequently asked questions and case studies offering guidelines and general advice for common developmental issues in children from birth to eighteen. The most important thing to remember is that each child follows their own unique path and that the unconditional love of a parent is the ultimate support a child can have on their journey of development.

Part 1
Learning to Move

1.
Motor Development in Babies and Young Children

In the womb

Many mothers can remember the joy of feeling their child move inside them for the first time. Sometimes it was a small kick, other times a tiny fist. While in the womb, babies move their head, torso, legs and arms. They react to sound and light through movement, discovering their surroundings – their sensorimotor development has begun. Babies will move more quickly if they hear loud noises, something mothers will undoubtedly notice and which may be a good reason to limit the amount of excitement in their surroundings. Mothers who have a healthy dose of movement during pregnancy help to stimulate movement in their unborn children.

Sensorimotor development is very complex. On an extremely simplistic level, we can summarise that our senses receive stimuli from our surroundings, which is processed and then prompts movement, i.e. our motor response. Movement and the information we receive through our senses are in constant interaction. Obviously, the nervous system is much more intricate than this, but for our purposes it's important just to remember that this sending and receiving is central to sensorimotor development.

Reflexes and early movement

After birth, babies have natural reflexes, such as sucking and grasping. Isn't it amazing how a newborn searches for its mother's breast and starts to drink, without even having opened its eyes? The grasping reflex is triggered as soon as something touches the palm of a baby's hand.

Soon, automatic movements appear, that is to say, movements that happen by themselves, for example balance, catching and self-support. However, it's important that these automatic movements are encouraged.

One of these automatic movements is the raising of the head. Four-week-old babies will try to raise their head if put on their stomach. This demands an enormous amount of energy and must be practised. Doctors recommend that babies sleep on their back in order to diminish the chance of sudden infant death syndrome (SIDS), so parents are understandably wary of placing babies on their front. However, if you are with your baby at all

Brainy babies!

A baby's first months are crucial. A baby's brain makes 700 new neural connections every second.[1] These connections form the foundations for sensorimotor development, as well as socio-emotional and language development, among others.

times, putting them on their front shouldn't cause a problem. Not only does the prone position strengthen head balance, but it also encourages complete physical development. This practice shouldn't be seen as a kind of training, but rather as a welcome change for babies from lying on their back.

The balancing reflex becomes active as soon as we lose our balance: muscle groups instinctively contract in order to regain stability. We support newborns completely when we pick them up, as they can't hold themselves upright yet. Babies slowly learn to control the muscle groups needed to stay balanced, eventually giving them enough confidence to learn to sit, stand and walk. Parents can stimulate the reaction for balance by encouraging activities that call for stability and steadiness, such as baby yoga and parent-and-baby swimming sessions.

The reflex to support oneself is also important. When babies' palms or foot soles are touched, they will extend their arms or legs. This teaches children that they can support themselves with their arms and legs. Children must dare to push themselves up so that they can eventually learn to stand.

When we fall, we automatically extend our arms to try and prevent injury. It's important that this reflex is practised sufficiently before a child learns to walk.

After approximately the first four months, these reflexes decrease and children begin to practise automatic movements. The first conscious movements now also take place, and children start to want to steer their own movements. It's always a wonderful moment when a baby consciously moves their hand towards an object and grabs it, or when a one-year-old beams as they stand on their own two feet for the first time.

Children who develop healthily learn from experience; they learn by doing. It's important that children's movements are in balance with their inner development. Motor development usually follows a certain pattern: rolling over, crawling, sitting and finally standing. By learning through experience, the child's foundation broadens. Each of these little steps contributes to the motor skills that form the basis of our lives.

While it's important that children practise movements, there should also be time for rest to process the experiences. Motor development demands time and space; it will happen automatically if the right conditions are in place. Hurrying the process simply doesn't work and disturbs the uniqueness of each child. Think about it this way: a two-year-old doesn't yet have the ability to skip; a five-year-old does.

If reflexes or automatic reactions aren't present in a child, or if motor development stops at a certain point, it's usually

TIP

Encouraging sensorimotor development in babies

▷ Lay babies on a firm surface on their back during their first months, followed by appropriate safe spaces thereafter, always with plenty of room to move. Offer them things to play with that they can grab and discover independently.

▷ Offer them toys of varying materials to encourage curiosity.

▷ Let children play undisturbed. Let them discover what they want to play with and how they want to play with it[2].

best to consult a professional, who will perform a series of developmental tests in order to find a root cause.

Developmental milestones: one step at a time

A popular child development principle is that of progressions from top to bottom (the cephalocaudal principle). Children first practise balancing their head on their shoulders, then learn to sit independently. Later, they learn to balance on two feet and eventually stand. Development also travels outwards, from torso to limbs (proximodistal development): children must first be able to sit firmly in a highchair before they can learn to use a spoon or fork. Another milestone is reached when children can bend over, demonstrating the required coordination between different muscle groups in order to keep balance. Isolated movement is the last step, for example intentionally moving only one finger or hand. Six-year-olds will often move their tongue from left to right when drawing. While it can just seem like a developmental quirk, this actually shows us what an enormous effort it is for them to perform the complex task at hand.

Not long ago, there were parents in my practice who proudly showed me that their six-month-old son could stand. They picked him up, put him on his toes and, with a little bit of support, the little boy could stand. However, the muscle reflexes on display here have nothing to do with the child actually balancing his weight on two feet and holding himself in the standing position. Children who develop in their own time and go through all the stages needed will eventually stand alone, and will be incredibly proud of themselves for doing so. Every parent will remember the moment their child stood unaided for the first time and what steps were taken to get to that point. It's always a wonderful moment when they finally succeed, at their own pace and in their own time.

Hand–eye coordination

I mentioned earlier that children's first conscious movement is usually grabbing with the hands. *Hand–eye coordination* is already present at birth, demonstrated when a newborn baby

TIP

Hand–eye coordination games

▷ While playing, children continually practise hand–eye coordination. Research has shown that babies prefer to look at a person's face, so talking and singing songs in view of babies are all highly engaging activities. Later on, you can add toys to heighten the experience.

▷ Have you ever heard of foot–eye coordination? Try drawing in sand with your big toe, or better still, draw with a pencil between your toes. Difficult, isn't it? You can develop this coordination by practising foot exercises, for example inching your foot forwards by curling and straightening your toes. This stimulation of the foot muscles should also be encouraged in children, so cuddle, massage and play games with your child's feet. If we connect strongly with our feet, we will stand more firmly on the ground.

grasps a finger and doesn't let go. However, it isn't until later that babies can open their hands fully, and later still that they're able to perform the pincer grip and hold an object between their thumb and forefinger (usually between eight and twelve months of age).

Rolling

A paediatrician refers Sarah to my physiotherapy clinic. Sarah is a sturdy fifteen-month-old girl who likes to sit with her legs slightly bent in front of her. From this position she plays with everything she can reach, but changes in pose such as rolling from her back to her front, or from her front to sitting, can only be performed with help. How can we support Sarah in her motor development?

After discussing the sensorimotor steps needed to move from lying to sitting and to standing with Sarah's parents, we then started looking for movement games and positions which would stimulate and challenge her. There are a number of positions that can be practised with children in this situation, starting with:

- The prone position – lying on the front. Let your child try this by laying them on their stomach for a short period of time while supervised. This is a stimulating position that encourages children to actively stretch their back, which is a prerequisite for the next motor step.
- Rolling over – this should only be done in a large playpen or on a soft carpet, but it can be seen as a child's

attempt at exploring their surroundings. It's also beneficial to the nervous system, particularly for the collaboration between the left and right hemispheres of the brain.

> **TIP**
>
> ## Rolling games
>
> Make a game of rolling over by lying down on the carpet with your baby (aged six months or older) and putting a toy just out of reach for them to reach for. You can use a noisy rattle, for example – anything to make the exercise fun and engaging for your child. Keep in mind that rolling over can still be a challenge for some toddlers and kindergartners, so for babies it's fine to adapt the game accordingly. You could loosely roll the child in a blanket, then challenge them to unroll it in order to free themselves. As always, keep in mind that exercises like this should be fun!

Crawling

Crawling is the next motor step, for which children must be able to support themselves on their hands and knees. Not only is crawling wonderful because children can move around independently for the first time, but they also gain experience in orienting themselves in the surrounding space – over the carpet, under a table, behind a box, to the right and to the left. This is a great incentive for the two hemispheres of the brain to work together. While crawling, the spine swivels back and forth, strengthening balance.

(TIP)

Encouraging crawling

▷ Provide incentives, such as toys just out of reach, or towers to topple.
▷ You can encourage your child by getting on all fours yourself and crawling with them over the bed, pillows, or floor. Just be sure to make a game of it!
▷ Make sure that the right conditions are present: for example, a soft carpet makes crawling easier than slippery polished parquet.

What happens if my child skips the crawling phase?

Many parents ask if skipping the crawling phase is bad for development. Opinions are divided on this subject, and while it's true that crawling provides an enormous impulse to sensorimotor development, it's worth keeping in mind that every child develops in their own way. But occasionally medical issues, such as problems with the hips, can be the reason a child doesn't crawl, so if you have any concerns do ask a professional. The following example comes from my own experience in my practice.

Sarah, the fifteen-month-old girl we talked about earlier, is a bum-shuffler. She moves across a smooth floor super-fast and can see everything around her. She even has her hands free, making it easy for her to grab things.

Shortly after birth Sarah had human respiratory syncytial virus (HRSV), a respiratory tract infection that causes babies to become short of breath. She was hospitalised and recovered slowly. This was an extremely distressing time for her parents. During her first year, she had regular colds, coughed a lot, tired quickly and was therefore weak, often crying. It was hard to keep her occupied, so her parents propped her up on pillows on the sofa or the floor. She received enough stimuli from the surroundings because she could see everything around her. Sitting caused her to get used to a single way of looking at the world, which is why she started to move around on her behind. She figured out that if she moved her legs in a certain way, she would move forward: bum-shuffling.

I gave her parents some tips, including the previously mentioned exercises to encourage rolling over. All the games were played in close proximity to her parents, for instance she rolled over their thighs while they sat on the floor. This way, she wasn't afraid to roll back and forth from her back to her stomach. Finding that different positions were safe, Sarah discovered whole new ways of moving and became increasingly active, even discovering crawling. Next Sarah started to walk on her knees, and from this position learned how to stand. Sarah was able to walk alone at two years of age, and although it took time and encouragement, she did it in her own way and with lots of fun.

Sitting

Children will usually learn to sit by themselves when they start to sit back while in the crawling position, using their hands to stay balanced. It's much better for a child's hips if they sit on their knees, rather than sitting on their bottom with their legs stretched out in front. You can help your child by sitting on the floor and supporting them between your legs while they sit on their knees. Rest against a wall or sit with a pillow behind your back if that's more comfortable for you.

Standing and walking

Children usually progress to the standing position by sitting on their knees and putting one foot on the ground in front of them. They pull themselves up and stand on wide-set, wobbly legs. And then comes the triumphant joy: I did it! I can stand! A slippery floor makes this much more difficult, which is

Should I prop my child up to encourage sitting?

Before your baby is able to sit unaided, having developed sufficient balance (around eight months), it isn't healthy to let them sit for more than a few minutes at a time. It could overburden the back as the muscles aren't yet strong enough to support it, and it isn't good for the development of the central nervous system.

If a child is put in the sitting position before they can sit by themselves, they won't take the challenge to crawl as readily, and will be more inclined to bum-shuffle, then pull themselves up into the standing position.

why bare feet or non-slip gripping socks are recommended.

Once children can stand, they will quickly begin to walk. While holding onto the sofa, coffee table or anything else in reach, they will slowly move forward on feet set wide apart. This is called a wide-based gait, giving more balance through a wider supporting surface. At first the entire foot is put down, but later the gait cycle is developed: moving from heel to the side of the foot to the toes.

Let your child practise on bare feet (as long as the floor isn't too cold) or in non-slip socks. Only after the first six months of walking are flexible shoes recommended. Walking is an incredible sensorimotor challenge, as the entire system has to work together to maintain balance. Standing upright and taking the first steps give both socio-emotional and cognitive development a great boost, as mobile children are more likely to notice and interact with their surroundings. Speaking will soon be next, and children will usually start to say their first words around this time: calling people and things around them by their names as well as communicating what they do or don't want.

TIP

Encouraging walking

▷ You can encourage children by walking together hand in hand, holding their hand as low as possible; or with a push-along toy, such as a trolley or cart, dolls' pushchair, or simple baby walker (not the sit-in kind).

▷ Walking is a rhythmical activity, so playing games that have rhythm can also help, for example singing games or counting while walking.

▷ Remember: just as every adult has their own walking pace, so does every child!

Communicating

Parents and children communicate both verbally and non-verbally from the very beginning of life. Talking to children is important for language development and learning to listen. Obviously, words are accompanied by gestures, intonation and mood, which is why motor development and learning to understand a language are so closely connected.

When children aren't quite at the speaking stage yet, it may be difficult for parents to understand what their child is trying to communicate. Using gestures or basic sign language encourages speech through movement, allowing children from six months and up to communicate before they can talk.

To be able to talk, a number of muscle groups have to work together in our tongue, larynx, neck, cheeks, lips and palate. Throughout motor development, muscles in the body are trained to work together and flex at the right moment: for example, children practise breathing while playing movement games, simultaneously developing their overall physical condition. This is why all the earlier phases, from lying on the stomach to learning to stand, provide the foundations of learning how to talk.

In my practice I often see misunderstandings occur when parents use

> **TIP**
>
> ## Encouraging talking
>
> ▷ Talking to babies is important for developing language and learning to listen. Talk to your baby from the very beginning of life.
>
> ▷ Using gestures or basic sign language encourages speech through movement, allowing children from six months and up to communicate before they can talk.
>
> ▷ You can find lots of resources online that provide more information on how to support your child's language development using non-verbal communication.

the words 'not' or 'none'. If you say to a child: 'Do not turn your cup upside down', the child doesn't register the word 'not' and understands that they should turn their cup upside down. This mixed-up thought process is also present in motor skills throughout the kindergarten phase and is evident in playground games of chase, in which the child who is evading capture might easily run right in front of the child who is 'it'.

Walking, talking and thinking are linked and are all essential parts of child development. Every child does things in their own good time, but children usually start talking by naming objects, animals and people. At age three or four, they begin to connect things and are able to think about their actions before they carry them out, for example: what should I do next? They can now also think about what's happened in their day.

The emergence of a dominant side

During the first few years of life, symmetrical and asymmetrical movements alternate regularly. During the first few months, a baby mostly moves asymmetrically. For

TIP

Helping to develop a sense of left and right

Left and right are abstract concepts. In daily life, we can help children learn these concepts by always starting to dress them from one of the two sides. For instance: first your right arm, then your left; first your right shoe, then your left. Or vice versa.

example, while one hand reaches to grab something, the other hand will not move. After that first phase, and until about four years of age, children mostly move symmetrically. For example, toddlers catch a ball with both hands. Not until children are around six years old will they demonstrate a preference or dominant side, i.e. their right or left hand. Children will

Right and left in young children

Watch the hands of very young children when they play: they will pick up a block that lies to their right with their right hand; if they want to lay it down to their left, they will switch hands to do so. The middle is a natural barrier. When a child no longer senses this barrier, a moment that often accompanies the development of a preferred side, the child is ready to draw from right to left, a prerequisite to learning how to write.

then consistently tend to hold their spoon with the dominant hand. We then also see an increase in complex movement such as walking and clapping at the same time, riding a bike or jumping over a rope.

Is my child a slow developer?

Sensorimotor development is spread out over many phases. If we remember that all children must learn to feel at home in their body and take their developmental journey at their own individual pace, we shouldn't look at motor development phases in black and white. No child will follow the charts in the exact week or month indicated for a specific phase of development, and they shouldn't be expected to.

The important thing is that children *continue* to develop. If you're worried about the motor development of your child, try keeping a diary or journal to document every new action or step taken. After a week, you may begin to notice that your child has made quite a lot of progress. Another possibility is to take a moment at the end of each day to reflect on what your child has done. How did they react to an event or stimulus? Were you surprised by their reaction, or did you notice any changes? If your child doesn't make significant steps in their motor development over a number of weeks, it's perhaps time to take a closer look with the help of a professional. Children who have been sick usually need time to catch up.

2.
Learning to Write

Should I give my five-year-old writing exercises?

Regular movement and focused practice can quicken motor development and perfect motor skills. However, it's important to keep to the appropriate skills for the child's phase of development, and not confuse continuous development with phased development. Although continuous development is, as it says, continuous, this doesn't necessarily mean that the more we put in, the more comes out. For example, if I were to spend a day practising skipping with a two-year-old, they would still

---

TIP

Choosing crayons and pencils

▷ Give two- to three-year-olds block crayons to work with.

▷ Give four- to six-year-olds thick stick crayons. At this age, the drawing movement is often still made with the whole arm.

▷ From six to seven onwards, if you want to challenge children to develop their fine motor skills, then they need to learn the correct pincer grip for holding a pencil. Giving them a triangular pencil can help. Thin, round pencils ask to be clutched or held incorrectly.

TIP

Physical exercises to prepare five-year-olds for writing

The following easy exercises help to prepare children of approximately five years of age for writing. The last exercise is for children of approximately six years of age.

▷ Stand firmly, swing your arms front to back simultaneously and then alternately.

▷ Take a long ribbon and create a large figure-of-eight shape by moving your arm in the air in front of you.

▷ Walk while swinging the ribbon in a figure-of-eight, forwards and backwards.

▷ Hold a stick in the preferred hand, move it up and down and twirl it.

▷ Try juggling. Learn the movement with one ball and practice later with two balls.

▷ Throw a tennis ball against a wall, let it bounce and catch it. Later, catch it directly without letting it bounce.

▷ Let a tennis ball bounce on the ground with one hand, keeping your palm faced downwards, but catching it with your palm faced upwards.

▷ Sit at a table with your feet on the ground. Lay your hand on the table palm up, then turn it palm down. Repeat with the other hand. Add finger exercises: touch the thumb to all fingers and repeat three times

▷ Test how many marbles you can pick up and put back with one hand.

▷ Practise a pincer-grip pencil hold with a pencil game. Try drawing exercises such as colouring, making straight lines and waves.

not have mastered the technique by the end of the day because their motor skills are not sufficiently developed to perform this complex movement.

The fine motor skills in most five-year-olds are not sufficiently developed to be able to make the complicated movements needed for writing. At this stage they still hold a pencil in their fist and move their arm from the shoulder, producing squiggles on the paper. The fine motor skills required for writing simply don't fit this developmental phase, and forcing the action before children are ready can have negative consequences.

In the second year of kindergarten (age five or six), most children are ready to learn to write the alphabet with a pencil. Giving an eight-year-old extra writing assignments to improve their handwriting makes sense, and practising with your child will improve their skills. But we have to be careful as parents and educators not to try and speed up the learning process by giving children exercises they aren't developmentally ready for.

How can I help my seven-year-old improve his handwriting?

The following is an example from my practice.

Jack is in first grade at school. The end of the year is near but, according to his teacher, he still writes much too slowly and messily. Jack is left-handed, reads above the average level and gets good grades in his other subjects. So why are his writing skills, and therefore his language skills, lagging behind? Jack comes into my practice with his school exercise book. The exercises are completed with pencil. The letters go every which way and are difficult to decipher. In order to analyse his handwriting, I give him a diagnostic test.

Jack immediately lets me know that he can't work on unlined paper. It strikes me that he doesn't differentiate between the size of letters and that he writes all over the page. His hand motor skills waver: he hesitates and rereads the text after every letter before he continues. If I ask him to read the sentence in full and then write it down, he writes without hesitating. Jack continually asks for confirmation that what he's doing is good. He writes slowly and with raised shoulders. I also notice that he blinks constantly. His mother continually asks if everything will be all right and reminds me that he's ahead of his peers in all his other school subjects. Next, we do a few finger exercises, which are often abandoned by schools after kindergarten, and then finish off by playing with a ball. I see that Jack finds it difficult to move with direction and his actions are somewhat uncontrolled.

We decide that the sessions shouldn't only be focused on writing and hand motor skills, but also on his gross motor skills. The most important thing is that the sessions are fun and that they allow Jack to learn to relax in his movements. I advise his mother to buy juggling balls and play together at home.

I also suspect that his poor writing results relate to him not being sufficiently challenged. Jack finds some exercises – tracing and copying – boring and he therefore does them without focusing. While working we pronounce the letters and sometimes draw them oversized in the air.

TIP

Practising finger dexterity

Children who steer their pencil from the shoulder will find it much more difficult to create a good result on paper. Children who need a bit more time for their sensorimotor development may experience pressure to perform if their school demands skills that have not yet been internalised, so be patient and encourage fun ways for your child to practise. The following will all help with finger dexterity and coordination, which are the prerequisites to writing skills:

▷ Finger games
▷ Crafts
▷ Modelling with clay
▷ Playing marbles
▷ Eating with a knife and fork

Jack immediately thinks up a story and begins to write it down, using the motor skills needed to write in a way that he enjoys. As we work, we reflect on what has been done, looking at and pronouncing every letter and word that he's written down correctly.

Part of the treatment is to make sure that his parents feel reassured, reducing any (unintentional) pressure Jack might feel at home and at school. Every child develops their motor skills in their own time. Certain skills are expected by mainstream schools, such as being able to draw the forms of letters around the age of five. These basic skills are needed for learning to write, but being able to hold a pencil in the correct way requires a very complicated

> **TIP**
>
> ### Encouraging good writing posture
>
> ▷ Posture while writing is very important.
> ▷ The paper should be straight in front of you, not askew, with the other hand on the table.
> ▷ Shoulders should be relaxed and beginner writers should loosen their arm after every sentence by shaking it at the side of their body and rolling the shoulders.

motor skill. Every child needs guidance in order to learn the correct grip. Children who can't grasp this technique yet will develop their own way of holding the pencil, such as clutching it in their fist and then drawing from the arm and shoulder. If the 'wrong' grip is learned, the correct one will have to be relearned when children start school. It's always so much more difficult to unlearn something that is ingrained than to learn it correctly the first time round.

In a world dominated by computers, is good handwriting important?

If your children go to a school that uses laptops regularly, make sure that they continue to practise writing. Writing is key to developing fine motor skills, and in high school (and later life) children need to be able to take notes quickly by hand; science subjects also require being able to write formulas legibly. I regularly work with high school children on improving their writing motor skills, because they were advised in primary school to do their homework on a laptop.

Part 2
Movement and the Senses

3.
Some Theory on the Senses

Our senses continually receive information about our body and the world around us. Mainstream medicine defines seven senses, of which the best known are hearing, smell, touch, taste and sight. The senses of balance and proprioception (the body's unconscious awareness of itself via sensory information) are less well known.

Anthroposophical medicine, however, recognises twelve senses, which operate across four different levels of the human being.

The four levels of the human being

When looking in detail at the way we function, it helps to divide human beings into the following four levels:

The physical body
This covers all the components of our actual body (cells, organs, limbs etc.), and all measurable and tangible physical reactions.

Life processes

This includes all the invisible physiological processes of the body that provide energy, enable us to grow, develop, heal and recover.

The soul

This refers to everything we experience: behaviour, feelings, thoughts and plans, both conscious and unconscious. Body and soul are easily distinguishable but inseparable. For example, on her birthday, a little girl runs around with rosy cheeks. The joy she feels is an experience of the soul, but is shown physically by running and laughing.

The *soul* expresses itself through the faculties of *thinking*, *feeling* and *willing*, which when combined determine our *behaviour*.

The 'I' or self

Soul and 'I' are seen as two different things. The soul is linked to behaviour and the 'I' signifies a person's spiritual core, what makes each person unique – their *individuality*, *identity* or *personality*.

The soul is the mediator between the spirit and the physical body. By using the soul, the spiritual core can express itself.

The twelve senses

Anthroposophy recognises twelve senses, which allow us to examine the way we function in more detail. These are divided into:

- four bodily (lower) senses
- four feeling (middle) senses
- four cognitive (higher) senses

The bodily senses

The lower senses of *touch, life, movement* and *balance* give the soul information about the body and pass information about the outside world inward. These bodily oriented senses form the foundation for sensorimotor development.

The feeling senses

Through the middle senses of *smell, taste, sight* and *warmth* children not only learn to recognise their surroundings but also their perception of these surroundings.

The cognitive senses

The four higher senses of *hearing, language, thought* and *ego* facilitate our spiritual qualities, allowing us to be our unique selves.

All of the above senses work closely together. The development of the four bodily senses forms the basis for the development of the feeling and cognitive senses. This approach highlights just how important the quality of experience is for a growing child's perception of the outside world. In order to feel at home in our body and in the world, the bodily senses must be well integrated.

4.
Touch – for Exploring and Feeling Safe

Through the sense of touch, children are able to experience their own body and explore the world. Babies first start to experiment with the sense of touch using their mouths. It's a constant battle making sure that nothing is eaten or swallowed! After six months the hands become an important way to feel and explore.

Does a dummy (pacifier) affect your child's sense of touch?

A dummy or pacifier can relax a crying child. However, babies first start to experiment with the sense of touch using their mouths. Using a pacifier too often can prevent children from using their mouth to develop their sense of touch. By putting objects in their mouth, children learn to identify objects and get to know their mouth, lips and tongue. If a baby sucks on a pacifier regularly, they miss out on these early sensory experiences.

The power of hugs

The skin is the most important organ for the sense of touch, providing the boundary between the inner and outer world. The sense of touch can only be experienced through boundaries: clothing, sheets, the sides of a cot or cradle.

The way children are lifted, carried and cared for is therefore very important. Hugs and cuddles not only give children intimate protection but also reinforce safe boundaries, both of which are desperately needed.

On an impromptu call to a friend's house, Tom, our friend's three-year-old boy, is excited by our unexpected visit. He runs back and forth in the room until his mother takes him on her lap and gives him a good hug. Slowly Tom relaxes, slides from her lap and goes to play quietly. This demonstrates the conscious act of a mother giving her child a hug so that he can connect with his body again through the sense of touch. Touching reinforces the feeling of safe boundaries and helps Tom to relax.

> **TIP**
>
> **Encouraging the sense of touch in young children**
>
> Giving young children many different types of toys encourages the sense of touch. Natural materials, such as water and sand, give endless hours of fun.

Massage for babies and children

Massage stimulates the sense of touch and lets children experience their own skin, reinforcing boundaries and giving a feeling of safety. Massage your baby after changing or bathing, and massage your toddler, kindergartener or schoolchild after their bath.

I often see children in my physiotherapy practice who have ice-cold hands and feet. These children sometimes have difficulty experiencing their bodies; massage and warm clothing can help them to strengthen this bodily connection.

(TIP)

Some tips for massage

▷ Use natural oils such as those from Weleda (see Resources). Calendula massage oils are often used when caring for babies.

▷ Make sure you have warm hands and a warm room.

▷ Take your time and make sure you're relaxed, otherwise you will pass your stress on to your child.

▷ It's best to massage using the palm of your hand, and make sure to adjust your movements to those of your child – they should be able to move with you.

▷ Moving your hands slowly will strengthen your own feeling experience and allow you to feel where your child's body is warmer or colder, and where the skin feels looser or tighter.

▷ Plan massage on a weekly basis, preferably on the same day and at the same time each week.

5.
Life – for Rhythm, Rest and Resilience

The anthroposophical sense of life (see p.39) tells us if we are comfortable. Small children can't voice this yet, but you can tell by their behaviour if they aren't.

The three Rs: Routine, Rhythm and Rest

Rhythm in every sense of the word enforces children's feelings of well-being and therefore influences the sense of life in a positive way. Rhythm gives structure and a foundation on which children can learn to move.

After birth, it's important that children find their own rhythm. The sleep–wake cycle and the feeding cycle slowly begin to develop in the first few weeks. The heart and breathing, as well as physiological processes such as digestion and metabolism, each have their own rhythm. 'Moving' in the right rhythm is of the utmost importance for growing children.

'Rhythm, rest and regularity', so well known but so difficult to enforce in our fast-paced lives, allow children to find their own rhythm. Parents often find keeping to the three Rs quite difficult, which is understandable in our

24-hour society, but knowing the importance of rhythm in raising children can help us to make better choices in our daily lives. A good night's sleep strengthens our sense of life and does wonders, even for parents!

Developing Rhythm

Rhythm and movement are connected, which is why it's so important that children experience rhythm inside and outside their bodies. Rhythmical movement is dynamic movement. But which movements are rhythmical? Crawling is rhythmical, and also helps children to start developing their own rhythm. Walking is rhythmical too. Going for a walk with a toddler, kindergartner or school child fits well with their natural rhythm. Research has shown that walking, at no matter what age, stimulates the brain and strengthens the entire system.

> **TIP**
>
> ### Again! Again!
>
> Rhythm can also be seen in the importance of repetition for young children, whether in playing games, singing songs or reading books. Parents will be familiar with cries of 'One more time!' Rereading a book, repeating a word or singing the same song every night at bedtime helps children to find and develop their own inner sense of rhythm, and strengthen their sense of life.

> ### What kind of music is most suitable for young children?
>
> ◆ Children's songs work best in four-four time, a simple marching rhythm (1, 2, 3, 4). Three-four time, a waltzing rhythm (1, 2, 3) isn't as suitable because children aren't yet able to move in time to the lilting beat.
> ◆ Recorded music played on a stereo or digital device is often much too fast for children to keep up with, and they literally run out of breath while singing!
> ◆ Rhythm is the basis for the development of language, so it's good for children to hear live music, which allows them to feel the beat and sing along, both at school and at home.

Which musical instrument would suit my child?

There are many things to take into account when choosing an instrument for your child. Musical instruments can be divided into the following general categories: woodwind (recorder, flute, clarinet), stringed instruments (violin, cello and guitar) and key/percussion instruments (piano and drums). Some instruments ask for more developed motor skills than others, and it may be that one in particular fits your 'type' of child. For this purpose, I would like to distinguish between three types of children: imaginative children, emotional children and doers.

The flute fits well with imaginative children, while stringed instruments suit emotional children, and doers prefer more earthly instruments such as piano and drums. Of course, this thinking isn't carved in stone, but you may find it a good starting point and it certainly worked in my own family. Keep in mind that the piano is a challenge for motor skills: two clefs to read and two hands playing different notes.

The appropriate age at which to start playing an instrument completely depends on the child's interests and capabilities. Children can start playing the piano or violin at age six, but a wind instrument is usually physically too difficult at that age. Some wind instruments require the child to have developed their adult front teeth before being able to play, and wind instruments require breathing stamina. Some music schools have open house days during which children can try different instruments, and if you as a parent play an instrument or you have one in your home, there's a good chance your child will become interested at an early age.

Does playing an instrument help with development?

Playing a musical instrument requires sensorimotor skills, concentration and perseverance and can significantly increase these qualitites. Research has shown that children who play an instrument have more 'learning capacity', and if they play in an orchestra, their listening abilities are increased dramatically as well.

How can I help my exhausted teenager?

The media often reports on the effects of too little movement in children. On the other hand, secondary school children, and even some children in the last years of primary school, can become overburdened by too many activities. Secondary school children often have tiring days,

Getting rid of a constant runny nose

All of life's processes have their own rhythm that together create energy. Our bodily systems have a great capacity for self-regulation and self-healing, and our immune system is stimulated and strengthened when faced with a challenge, such as a virus or a cold. It's important that time is taken for the recovery process. Research has shown that in the first years of life our immunity is strengthened when given the chance to overcome minor illnesses on its own. Therefore, perhaps it is worth giving children the rest they need to recover from colds instead of giving medication at the first signs of discomfort.

especially if the trip to and from school is long. Many sport clubs ask that children practise two to three times per week and play matches at the weekend. This can be too much for adolescents: their bodies become depleted, resulting in slow growth and exhaustion.

Hannah is referred to me for physiotherapy by a paediatrician. She has seen all kinds of doctors because of continuous headaches and fatigue but no one has been able to help her. She is fourteen years old and is working towards her exams. She has a busy home life, helping to care for her mother, who is in a wheelchair. She sounds desperate and disappointed. She has missed lots of school because of her condition, even being admitted to hospital for observation for a couple of days, and her fatigue is stopping her from having an active social life. Hannah is extremely motivated and really wants to get back to school, but her biggest downfall is overestimating what she can and can't do.

Together with the school, we set up a roster so that she can attend school but only for a certain number of hours a day for the first couple of weeks. Her father takes her to school with her bike in the boot so that she only has to cycle home. After three months of physiotherapy sessions, Hannah doesn't yet go to class every day but is riding her bike to and from school. As much as she would like to do more, it's important that she keeps her current ability in mind. A few weeks later we round the physiotherapy sessions off. Hannah still has headaches but they're much less disruptive and she's learned how to deal with her fatigue better, even seeing her friends outside of school again. Now, Hannah comes to me every winter. She's back at school and her headaches and fatigue have stopped, and one yearly physiotherapy session gives her all the support she needs.

Hannah presented a relatively severe case of exhaustion, but the solution in cutting back on activity to an appropriate degree and taking essential rest is relevant to all cases.

6.
Movement –
for Healthy Activity

Earlier we said that motor development shouldn't be hurried through over-practising. Motor development is a maturation of the motor system as early reflexes are phased out and motor movement becomes much more complex. Children practise movement constantly, and as they get older their movements become more controlled and purposeful, much like the way a rider learns to steer a horse. The most important thing is that children develop their sense of movement in their own time and in their own way. Moments of rest are a must, as they provide an opportunity to internalise development.

The sense of movement isn't only concerned with the movement of the body, but also with movement in our surroundings. For instance, imagine a five-year-old letting a ball bounce and trying to catch it. She holds her arms slightly apart, determined by the sense of movement. The first few times, the ball may bounce too softly or too hard and the child doesn't hold her hands in the right place to catch it. She will adjust the strength and placement of her arms and react to the movement of the ball. In doing so, the child is reacting to a movement outside herself in order to catch the ball. Anticipating movement outside of our own bodies is an important, but often underestimated, part of the sense of movement.

Our sense of movement can also provide a lot of pleasure and a feeling of freedom. I remember being four years old and climbing up onto a high sand dune. The experience of feeling the warm sand under my feet, in which I sometimes sunk deeply, and climbing on all fours until I was at the top gave me an enormous sense of pleasure. This is the pleasure of the sense of movement and is a wonderful experience for every child. Emotions and experiences belong in the soul. My soul was willing me to reach the top of the dune and in order to realise this, I began to move. But there is also a 'spiritual' aspect to this unique experience that anchors it so firmly in my memory. You could say that a child doesn't just 'grow up' to reach their goals, but also 'grows inwards' to achieve them.

Why is my child so clumsy?

A mother who called to make a physiotherapy appointment for her six-year-old son told me, 'My son, Oliver, is so clumsy. He always seems to trip over things, and doesn't want to play with other children or play football. We decided it would be best for him to stay in kindergarten for another year instead of moving up to first grade.'

Describing a child as clumsy is a rather bold statement and can be hurtful. The word 'clumsy' is a negative word, and doesn't describe the child but the way he moves. This is one of the reasons why I try not to have children in the same room when I speak to parents about their worries in initial interviews. Speaking about children while they're in the room isn't pleasant and may even be detrimental to their well-being. A test to assess the level of motor development, relative to the child's age, is always the first step after establishing parents' or educators' concerns. This type of test not only gives me an indicative score but also shows me how the child performs certain motor tasks.

In Oliver's case, we made an appointment for him to come and see me. Oliver, a sturdy boy quite big for his age, steps into the room

> **Practice makes perfect!**
>
> For a child, physical clumsiness means that they have developed a strategy not to participate in activities that highlight their lack of motor skills, i.e. don't play tag, because you will always be 'it'. Unfortunately, this also means that they get less chance to practice these motor skills, which is actually what they need to improve: they will learn through repetition and practice. Having fun while practising creates a positive experience.

with curiosity. I ask him to do a few activities to see what his motor skills are like. For each task, Oliver needs to take time and have a few tries before being able to plan his movements. For example, one of the tasks is to bounce a tennis ball against the wall, let it bounce on the floor once and catch it. The first time, he throws too hard for it to bounce. Then he throws too softly. He tries to throw underhand but the ball hits the ceiling instead of the wall. I show him how to throw overhand and, after three tries, he's able to catch the ball ten times in a row.

I decide on the following treatment goal: to make Oliver feel enthusiastic and confident about his own motor abilities. With Oliver's parents, we decide that after completing

Put your own shoes on!

Many young children can't learn to tie their shoelaces because they are bought shoes with zippers or velcro, and if they do have lace-up shoes, their parents will tie their laces for them. This might save time in the short term, but doesn't help children, who need to learn through doing and practice.

our physiotherapy sessions, he will choose a sport that he would like to play and that suits him. It's always wonderful to see how enthusiasm diminishes constraints, even in Oliver's mother, who was rightfully worried about her son. Only a few weeks after starting the sessions, Oliver is meeting up with his friends after school and, after having taken a trial lesson, has chosen to attend judo classes.

Every child's sensorimotor development is unique. It isn't about forcing, but about creating enthusiasm. It's also about setting an example and giving the right instructions on how to perform a motor skill, then allowing children to practise and repeat what you demonstrated.

Which kind of sport would suit my child?

Parents regularly ask me which sport best fits their child. Playing a sport at a young age is often encouraged – some three-year-olds already have swimming badges, and at four they're on the football field. However, is such specific training good for young children? If the sport is given in the form of play, then it fits the developmental phase of young children. Once the play changes to competition, it doesn't belong there any more.

More and more children are participating in sports, which in itself a positive development. However, it's also true that the percentage of young children who have injuries caused by physical exertion has similarly increased. I often treat children who have sport injuries. Could this have something to do with pressure to perform?

Below I have described a number of sports in order to give some general advice on which sport might best fit which child. I have chosen sports that tend to be the most popular and have taken for granted that all of these sports are undertaken in the form of play. I seriously recommend that parents attend the first few practice sessions with their child to see how the instructor or coach works with children. When considering these activities from a sensorimotor viewpoint, it's important to see how complicated the motor skills needed for the sport are. Can your child do what is asked?

What if my child is not 'sporty'?

If you don't think your child is suited to 'mainstream' sports, remember that there are lots of other activities such as theatre, eurythmy (a form of purposeful movement combined with speech and music, and taught in Steiner-Waldorf schools, see p.68) and free dance that require creativity as well as movement. There's bound to be an activity your child really enjoys, even if it takes a few tries to find the right one.

Swimming

Swimming is symmetrical. Arms and legs must move simultaneously and so this activity is best suited to the symmetrical phase (age six and up). Simultaneously but independently moving arms and legs asks for developed motor skills and takes quite some practice. Children need energy to grow, but swimming lessons, especially when taken twice a week, ask for a lot of energy. I often hear parents complain that their kindergartner is tired or has a cold or an ear infection regularly due to swimming lessons. Stomach aches caused by taking in chlorinated water are also commonplace. It's therefore important for parents to decide at what age they allow their child to start swimming lessons. Children aged six years and older master the technique of swimming much quicker than younger children. However, even if a young child has achieved a number of swimming certificates or badges, they still don't have enough insight into their own capabilities while swimming and will need constant supervision.

Football

If your child can stand on one leg (and will therefore not fall over when kicking a ball) and they can share and play together with other children, then they should be able to enjoy a football club or group. Young children often kick the ball with both left and right feet and have great fun while running over the field. Keep in mind that regular practice sessions and weekend matches ask for very one-sided movement, which can cause injuries.

Tennis

The sensorimotor skills needed for tennis are complicated. Children need to have developed a preferred hand to hold a racket. Tennis requires asymmetrical movement, while anticipating the ball and judging speed need a certain kind of insight. Even following the coach's instructions requires a lot of concentration. With this in mind, I advise parents not to enrol children in tennis lessons until they are seven years of age. It goes without saying that only when children meet the above requirements will they be able to enjoy playing tennis. The need for complicated motor skills that are above a child's ability can be the reason why they stop enjoying a certain sport.

Riding

The best age to start horse riding is between six and eight. The most important prerequisite is that your child can follow directions and understand that horses are flight animals and can be frightened by sudden movements. Children should therefore first learn to handle and be around ponies or small horses, getting to know the animal through contact and taking care of it. Many young children dream of riding horses, but it requires considerable concentration, and the abilities to give focused direction to movement and to focus their will.

Balance and the coordination of arms and legs can be stimulated by riding, as well as correct posture, which in turn strengthens the back and stomach muscles. Over the years I have seen many children, especially older children and adolescents, improve their balance and strength through horse riding.

Young children usually ride small ponies so that they don't have too far to go if they fall off, but a good riding cap and breeches will help prevent most injuries. It's also good to research stables with licences and safety certificates to make sure they satisfy the necessary requirements.

Ballet and gymnastics

For the sake of convenience, I will discuss ballet and gymnastics together as they have many similarities. In general, children feel freer when dancing, and ballet and gymnastic exercises can help to strengthen the muscles used for good posture. However, both classical ballet and gymnastics ask quite a bit from our musculoskeletal system. Children are coached to stand with a hollow back, which might influence their posture in daily life. Stretching, needed for some of the exercises, should be done under strict guidance and without pain. The coach should also keep in mind that children don't always dare to speak up if something hurts. Once an element of competition is added, children want to perform well and don't want to disappoint their parents or coach. It's these children that I see in my practice: children with back pain, ankle or knee injuries, or dislocated shoulders, all incurred while doing gymnastics. If children compete at a high level, there's usually enormous pressure to get them back on track after an injury. For this reason, it's extremely important that muscle strength and coordination are the focus during recovery and before practice is resumed.

Avoiding sports injuries

Children love playing sports and moving about. But sometimes they hit a wall: their own physical barrier. These are the children who come for physiotherapy.

Jasper is seven. He goes to football practice twice a week and plays a match every weekend. Jasper stumbles

---

Sports injuries – when to see a doctor

- Most physical injuries in children occur through falling or being pushed, causing minor bruises and sprains. If a child can't stand on a leg because of excessive pain, it's time to consult a doctor.
- Minor injuries usually heal within three weeks. If it takes longer, I would advise a visit to your GP.

---

into the room when he comes to see me at my clinic. His legs hurt. Where? 'Everywhere,' he says. During the physical examination, it becomes evident that the tendons of certain muscle groups are especially sensitive. He's been taking painkillers for a month so that he can continue playing, but now he's just in too much pain.

This is *overexertion*. Children who are growing are particularly susceptible to overexertion. The reason for this is that their bones grow faster than their muscles. Often children start complaining of soreness after a growth spurt: when the bones have grown, the muscle system is out of balance and the muscles are too short. If these muscles are used too much, the tendons can become irritated and begin to hurt. Rest is the best medicine for overexertion. As a physiotherapist, I also look at the child's posture and muscle coordination.

As Jasper's case shows, a six- to seven-year-old can't pinpoint pain yet – it's everywhere. However, although the pain experience can be quite high, I don't believe that giving painkillers is the right thing to do. Children must learn to experience their 'boundaries', including their pain

> **TIP**
>
> ### Choosing sports shoes
>
> Good sports shoes are a must. Shoes should fit well, have a sturdy heel and arch support, and the laces should be tightly tied.

threshold. Pain means STOP!

In general, this type of injury takes six weeks to heal. Six weeks with no football is torture for a football fanatic like Jasper, so we decide to work on muscle coordination and balance for four weeks. After this, he's allowed to slowly start practising again and after six weeks he can play his first match. A big advantage is that he notices his technique has improved!

7.
Balance – for Strength and Poise, Inside and Out

Physical balance

Balance is a miraculous thing. By lifting their head, holding it still, sitting and finally standing upright, children conquer gravity. Naturally, the sense of balance is closely connected to the sense of movement, but as humans, we only learn to stand upright because of the behaviour of those around us. Children directly observe us as adults and imitate, which means it's incredibly important that we set a good example, even in our movements.

> **TIP**
>
> ### Sitting 'properly' at the table
>
> You should regularly check whether the proportions of chairs and tables at home and at school are still correct, especially after a growth spurt.

Every child stands upright when they're ready. Some children have to practise endlessly by shuffling along while holding onto the sofa. Others stand, wobble and sit back down until they finally figure it out and can quite suddenly stand up and walk without holding on. Most likely due to her difficult start, Sarah (the super-quick bum-shuffler

> ### TIP
> ### Games for balance skills
>
> Playground and party games such as Red Light, Green Light and Musical Statues can encourage and develop children's sense of balance.
>
> ▷ One child stands at one end of the playground/ room with her back to those at the other end.
> ▷ When ready, the child shouts 'Green Light!' and the group runs towards her.
> ▷ When the child shouts 'Red Light!', everyone has to freeze.
> ▷ If you're still moving, you're 'it'.
> ▷ Suddenly having to freeze always proves a fun but tricky challenge for the sense of balance! You can practise the same skills at home by playing Musical Statues.

from earlier, pp.21–24) didn't stand alone until she was around two years old.

Children first walk straight ahead, while directions in space – left, right, ahead, behind, below and above – become integrated in the system of movement over time. Becoming one with a movement and letting it connect with our own experience and purpose is a complex process in time and space.

Why is good balance important?

I often see children in my practice who have developed a strategy to cover up their poor sense of balance. Tasks are done hastily and things are dropped 'on purpose'. These children usually sit on the floor when they put on or take off their shoes as it provides the necessary support. If children are unsure of their balance, this is often reflected in their motor skills.

Torso balance is a prerequisite for eating with a fork and spoon, drawing and learning to write, so encourage your child to sit straight and on two buttocks while at the table. A straight back helps with balance and prevents future back problems.

TIP

Checking back strength and mobility

Here are some ways to check whether children have enough mobility in their back to stand or sit straight:

▷ Children should be able to reach the ground with their hands when bending forwards while keeping their legs straight.

▷ Children should be able to lift themselves back into a straight position with their hands placed on their neck while keeping their back straight.

▷ Ask children to sit on the ground with their legs straight out in front of them. Can they bend as far forwards as they can backwards?

Nature and spatial awareness

A lot of research is currently being done on the human brain and the body's spatial awareness. One particular study recently showed that children who grow up in Indian Sanskrit schools could indicate north, south, east and west precisely. Even inside a classroom, 87% of the children still

Playing in nature

Any movement that challenges a child's feeling of balance also stimulates the sense of balance. Natural playgrounds in which children can climb trees and scramble over slippery trunks or rocks are much more challenging than standard playgrounds. All the senses are stimulated when playing in nature. A lot of research has been done on the effects of playing in green spaces, and has shown that children who play in natural playgrounds develop better sensorimotor skills. Not only do natural environments work positively on motor development, but children also score higher on skills such as self-confidence and the ability to play together.

knew which direction was which when asked.[3] Through their education and upbringing these children have an intense connection with their environment. They can distinguish between eight compass points and they know the position of the Sun. Similar research in school children in Switzerland showed that not one of them knew which way was north or south when inside. Experiencing the environment, for example knowing the position of the Sun, helps us to experience time and space, which explains why going out and exploring the environment is a must for children. Tending a vegetable garden together or even taking a daily walk around the block while looking at the changes that have occurred over time strengthen children's connection with their surroundings.

Can I improve my child's spatial awareness?

When discussing sensorimotor development, I described how we acquire spatial awareness through movement. When a child stands up, they're free to move in all directions: to the left, to the right, a step ahead, look up or down, climb. Walking backwards asks for extra skills and trust. Many children (and adults) still look back when walking backwards. The sense of movement together with the sense of balance form the foundations for being able to orient ourselves in space.

Imaginative play is excellent for sensorimotor development. Through peekaboo and playground games, role-playing and verses accompanied by movement, children learn to be in command of their body and strengthen their spatial awareness. For example: how many steps is it to the other side? Can I still tag him? Children learn through exploring, by doing.

Inner balance and resilience

How can I help my child become more resilient?

'Resilience' in children is a much-cited concern among parents, usually focused on their child's social or emotional vulnerability.

When a three-year-old gets upset because his toy has been snatched by another child, this has nothing to do with being 'resilient' – this is appropriate to the young child's developmental stage. 'Resilience' in children shouldn't even be discussed until they are halfway through primary school.

A mother has asked me to see her son, Luke, because

Learning to share

Finding balance is hard work, from moving around and standing, to gaining the inner balance and self-awareness to say 'I' around the third year. When inner balance is accomplished, children can start to share. This isn't possible until children have first experienced their own space; only then can they open up to let someone else in, for example, by sharing their toys with another child.

he's clumsy and doesn't behave well socially. He's been referred for special needs support by his school. I gave Luke physiotherapy when he was in first grade to help him with his writing skills. Luke asked his mother if he could come back to me before seeing the special needs teacher in case physiotherapy helped, and she agreed.

Luke, now nine years old, timidly enters the room. I notice that he walks slightly hunched over, with slumped shoulders. He looks down when he shakes my hand and says hello. While we talk he constantly pushes his glasses up on his nose. This description gives us an idea of who Luke is. We could categorise him as a non-resilient child. However, his physical demeanour tells us nothing about his rich inner world. Not only does Luke know a lot, he's enormously eager to learn and thinks about the world a great deal. He's aware of his gift. He explains, 'First I think for a minute, weigh up the pros and cons, and then my reaction is always too late.' This delayed reaction isn't accepted socially. Luke has become stuck and sees himself as physically and socially incompetent.

Feeling free and safe in their own body should be the starting point for every child. Luke worked on various exercises for several weeks to train his motor skills and assertiveness, including ones inspired by Sherborne developmental movement therapy and the Rock and Water programme (see below). He loved them and they encouraged him to start working on his posture by himself, which helped him stop the tic with his glasses. He started to make play dates again and was able to sleep through the night. It appeared that this approach was enough to untangle the knot of stress that had surrounded Luke.

> *TIP*
>
> ## Quality of sleep helps assess inner balance
>
> Assessing whether children are getting regular, quality sleep is a good way to tell if they are in harmony with themselves and their surroundings.

Movement techniques and therapies

The Sherborne approach is a developmental movement therapy in which movements are turned into physical games between parent and child, allowing them to share experiences, which strengthens the child's physical, social and thinking skills.

Originally developed in the Netherlands to support young men and boys with behavioural problems, Rock and Water is an exercise programme that combines social skills, sport and movement activities. Developing physical resilience isn't the only goal, but also the path to the development of confidence and social skills (social, psychological and spiritual identity).

Bothmer Gymnastics is a series of specially developed movement exercises that was introduced in the first Waldorf School in Stuttgart (1919). Intending to develop both inner and outer balance, the approach focuses on using movement to explore the body's relationship with space and direction, as well as encouraging confidence and coordination. It's widely taught in Steiner-Waldorf schools, with exercises tailored to the developmental needs of each age group.

Eurythmy engages the entire body, soul and spirit in focused movement. It is commonly used in Steiner-Waldorf schools to support child development. Eurythmy teachers help pupils to develop graceful and purposeful movement through exercises, patterns and activities that use movement, music and speech, which increase in complexity over their school lives based on age and ability. Eurythmy is a fantastic way to increase a child's sense of spatial awareness and orientation, and is also used as a form of movement therapy in anthroposophical medicine to restore balance to the body after illness.

8.
The Feeling and Cognitive Senses

The bodily senses covered so far in Part 2 – of *touch*, *life*, *movement* and *balance* – all clearly form part of sensorimotor development, but they also form the foundation for the feeling and cognitive senses. However, the twelve senses (see pp.39–41) all work closely together simultaneously throughout life. Broadening children's experience through tasting different foods, playing with a range of objects and materials, looking at picture books full of colourful illustrations, naming what they see in the books, and parents reading to them all contribute to their development and the overall aim of becoming rounded, confident individuals who will be able to think clearly and creatively.

The feeling senses – smell, taste, sight and warmth

Of the four feeling senses, *smell*, *taste* and *sight* are the most well known, but anthroposophical medicine also recognises the sense of *warmth*. All four of these senses are connected to our surroundings and our personal experiences. By activating them through a variety of stimuli we can also encourage sensorimotor development.

> **TIP**
>
> **Cold hands and feet**
>
> Make sure that your child's hands and feet are nice and warm in the winter with good quality woollen gloves and socks. Many children have difficulty determining this themselves and only realise their own hands are cold when they hold a warm one.

For example, by providing fresh food with many different *tastes*, we stimulate the sense of taste and broaden children's experience of food and therefore their personal preferences.

Sight gives a great deal of support to balance, so much so that a ten-year-old may not want to stand with his eyes closed for fear of falling over.

The sense of *warmth* may not be so well known, but it's hugely important and absolutely essential for sensorimotor development.[4] This sense doesn't only encapsulate physical warmth, but also the warmth of a friendly encounter. Enthusiasm is an important expression of warmth and human involvement.

The cognitive senses – hearing, language, thought and ego

The cognitive senses – *hearing, language, thought* and *ego* – reveal an individual or 'intentional' side of the senses. However, in order to determine the intention of an impulse, children must have reached a certain level of physical and soul development.

The following is an example of the sense of *hearing*. Imagine you call your child by their name. The child hears their name but also hears you. They will not only react to recognising their name but also to your tone, the volume at which you call them, as well as to your demeanour and any gestures you use.

At first the sense of *language* only exists rudimentarily. Depending on where a child is born, they will learn one or more languages with which to name the things in their world. The sense of speech allows us to listen and know: is this about me? Does this affect me? It's therefore important that adults speak well, pronouncing words and sentences clearly and correctly.

It's also important for the sense of speech that the sense of movement is able to develop in its own way and at its own speed. By moving intentionally with the help of games, rhythm, lots of repetition and moments of rest, the sense of movement is stimulated directly, while the sense of speech is also encouraged. The conversion of movement into speech takes place continually by adults naming things and children experiencing them through movement.

Why reading matters

The power of learning language and words in child development can't be underestimated. As an author of children's books, I often tell pupils about the effect of reading while visiting schools. If children read for fifteen minutes a day, they will learn 1,000 new words a year. A child also learns about 1,000 words per school year, so by doubling this amount through reading, the vocabulary expands enormously, which supports the capacity to think.

The sense of *thought* stands for both interpreting someone else's thoughts and learning to think for yourself. Children are not able to form their own thoughts until around three years of age. The sense of thought is formed through the enormous amount of information children see, hear and experience. Language serves thought, so the more words and language we offer our children, the more opportunities they have to develop their sense of thought.

The *ego*, or sense of 'I', of individuality, develops by us experiencing ourselves in relation to others, and is supported through loving, trusting relationships.

9.
Overstimulated and Hyperactive Children

Processing sensory information

The combination of the senses and reacting to the information that these senses give (i.e. doing) is called *sensory processing*. A number of unconscious steps must be taken before we can actually 'do' something:

1. *Observing*, which is carried out by the senses: you hear the sound of a young child crying while you're at a busy playgroup.
2. *Orientation*, or 'finding our bearings': you focus on the observation. As a parent, if you hear a child crying you immediately react and think: 'Do I recognise this sound, is it my child?'
3. *Interpreting*: you recognise your child's cry but know that it's more whining than crying, and your child is probably just tired.
4. *Organising*: you go to your child to check that your interpretation was right.
5. *Acting* on your reaction: you pick your child up and comfort him.

Sensory processing develops as children grow, have more experiences, and learn from them. Children who are highly sensitive may react strongly to stimuli that they feel are too much (such as seams in socks), while other children are the complete opposite (they may have a blister but don't feel any pain while they are playing; they don't notice anything until they stop and sit down). Good sensory processing is a prerequisite for alertness while playing, learning and discovering.

If this process is 'disrupted', such as in the case of children with a mental or physical disability, the child will automatically avoid stimuli or drown them out, which causes stress. Another possibility is that children don't take on stimuli at all. Investigation into how the sensory process is being disturbed is then needed in order to support and help the child in their development.

Is my restless baby overstimulated?

Learning to process information via the senses slowly develops during the first years of life, but it is gradual and it's important to control babies' environments so they don't become overloaded with sensory stimuli. Providing babies with a regular routine, including particular times for feeding, changing and sleeping, can help with this. When babies' developing senses are given too much information to process, such as loud noises, bright lights or being moved too quickly, they become overstimulated. There's a reason why we tiptoe into a baby's room! Overstimulation can result in restlessness both when awake and when sleeping. By giving the baby the three Rs – routine, rhythm and rest – they will sleep more deeply and for a longer period of time. A sling in which the baby's back is supported in a gently curved position can also help them to sleep more comfortably.

A nap during the day is important for toddlers, as is a period of rest for kindergarteners. Even teenagers still need time to themselves to recharge their batteries. At any age, children's resilience is directly related to how they feel. When children feel relaxed and rested, they will be able to react much better to changes in their environment than if they are tired.

How can I help my hyperactive child calm down?

Some children are highly sensitive. They register everything around them and their senses become overwhelmed, including their sense of movement, preventing them from being able to effectively experience or steer their own movements. In other words, they become hyperactive. However, if you focus on solving the problem through exerting control, they will only become frustrated. Many parents will know all too well that you can't make a hyperactive child sit still on a chair for a long period of time – it simply doesn't work. But there are experiences that can show your child how to take command and control of their own movements.

Children need space to let go, so physical and rhythmical activities can be beneficial (see pp.54–58 for my tips on choosing a sport for your child, and pp.47–48 for tips on selecting a muscial instrument). Anything that helps children to take command of their body and their movements will result in calmer and more focused behaviour. Always make sure that the activity suits your child and is appropriate for their age and stage of development.

10.
Why Cut Down on Screen Time?

The digital world, television, computers and phones all influence a child's movement (or lack of it). Research has shown that children have exchanged time traditionally spent moving and playing outside for 'digital' time, during which they are usually physically passive, often moving only a single finger while playing on a touch-screen device. Children don't activate their system during 'digital' time – in other words, they aren't creating new neural pathways. If young children only move, play and jump around virtually, we should ask ourselves what kind of mental movement qualities they will develop. How will they move as social thinkers or as loving human beings when they are adults?

If we take this problem seriously, we as parents and educators should come to no other conclusion than that our growing children must cut down on their 'digital' time. Young children can't do this alone and adolescents have extreme difficulty in sensing where their boundaries lie. They need adults to help them. In recent years there has been extensive research on the influence of the use of digital devices[5] and you can find recommended books on how to approach the topic of screen time on pp.95–97.

Can playing video games cause back problems?

Children now not only move too little, but often don't move correctly. Medical specialists report that more and more children (nicknamed the 'Gameboy generation') complain of back and neck pain because they spend too long sitting hunched over their tablets and smartphones. The term 'text neck' has even been added to medical jargon.[6]

I regularly see children who come to my practice complaining about severe headaches, neck and back pain. What strikes me again and again is that many children have no idea about their own posture. As long as they don't feel pain in their limbs or back they have no idea if they are standing up straight or hunched. Usually it's the parents who are worried and raise the alarm. Many healthcare systems don't do much when it comes to prevention, although some schools do make the effort to provide ergonomic chairs in classrooms.

Between eleven and fourteen years of age, most children experience a growth spurt. This is the age when heavy schoolbags full of books and laptops are carried, but also tends to be the age of slouching on the sofa. But it isn't just this kind of activity that

> **Tip**
>
> ### Encouraging good posture
>
> To help improve your child's posture, ensure that when sitting at the table, their back is straight and their feet are planted firmly. Sitting actively, that is without leaning against the back of the chair, strengthens the back muscles. Place any computers or tablets on a platform, such as a thick book, so that your child can remain sitting straight without having to bend their neck.

can hinder good posture: doing homework while sitting with a laptop or tablet on the lap strains both the back and neck muscles. This in turn can lead to the development of an abnormal stance in the hips or knees, resulting in an ungainly walk or difficulty when running. In the long term, this can result in joint degeneration of the hips and knees. Simply telling a child to 'sit up straight' usually doesn't help because children physically no longer know how to and don't have the stamina to keep it up.

Is playing active video games as good as playing outdoors?

My husband and I volunteer with disabled children at a local social project in which the children develop and care for a vegetable garden. Last week, we sowed beets with the children. Some of them used gardening equipment but most preferred to work with their hands in the earth. They prepared the seedbed perfectly, after which each seed was carefully placed in the ground and covered with a bit of earth. The way they did this, so carefully, with utter respect and full of concentration, touched me.

Practising purposeful movement, such as that used in eurythmy (see p.68), may seem obvious, but so many movements these days – for example, active computer games in which children move by kicking a virtual ball – have no tangible purpose. Yes, this activity involves movement, but it's pretence – it isn't paired with movement by the soul or 'I'. Many of these consoles and games are promoted as being a remedy against the lack of movement in children. However, research has shown that they don't have a lasting effect on the amount of time children spend moving: as soon as the game stops, the child stops.[7] While movement should be encouraged, we can only guess what effect this kind of 'virtual' movement and experience has on the well-being of children and adults in the real world.

Part 3
Movement and Learning

11.
Learning through Movement at Every Age and Stage

Learning through living

Learning has become an abstract process in many schools. Children sit and work, and are not given sufficient opportunities to develop key sensorimotor skills. The close relationship between movement and experience, or 'learning through living', can be seen in a number of schooling systems around the world, but Steiner-Waldorf schools in particular pay special attention to learning through movement. For example, in cooking lessons children learn about abstract concepts such as weight when measuring sugar and flour. Here, the principle of 'learning through living' is practised by learning through *meaningful* experiences. Through positive experience, enthusiasm is kindled and children's will is stimulated – they want to learn – providing them with the best possible outlook for learning.

But this principle doesn't have to be confined to 'practical' subjects. A study performed by the University of Groningen in the Netherlands found that combining learning with movement in the classroom can give better school results. A programme called 'Fit and Skilled' was developed in which children moved energetically for half an hour three times a week during maths and language lessons. Scientists found that walking and jumping caused the children's brains to release adrenaline, enabling information to be absorbed more effectively – illustrating the undeniable link between movement and learning.

Abstract concepts are much easier for children to understand if they are accompanied by movement, or *doing*. For example, for a child to understand that five apples are greater than two, they must first learn to count using their fingers, beginning with one hand and then progressing to both. This is the basic foundation for learning the essentials of arithmetic. Learning to 'grasp' abstract numbers and quantities with our fingers in this way causes a neural connection, and research has shown that young children with nimble fingers are able to learn arithmetic skills more easily later on.[8] Finger games are important for developing this ability, while playing a musical instrument can also be a wonderful stimulus for hand dexterity.

In Ancient Greece, sensorimotor learning was applied by rhythmically walking while memorising a poem, and today, research proves that our memory functions at its best when we move while speaking out loud, enabling us to create the all-important neural pathways needed for learning and development. Using repetitive movements such as walking and counting sounds simple, yet in my experience I have come across many children who have great trouble in stepping or jumping while counting at the same time. Walking and counting backwards simultaneously is even more difficult. This gap in ability demonstrates that the child has not yet achieved freedom of movement (insufficient motor maturation), and that this particular skill needs more attention. There are lots of ways to encourage this connection: for example, activities such as circle games allow children to establish and practise this neural link, especially if they are accompanied by counting exercises.

Do boys and girls learn and develop differently?

The first seven to eight years of life are vital to the development of the brain as lots of neural pathways are created during this time. The left hemisphere of the brain grows more slowly than the right hemisphere. The hormone testosterone intensifies this process in boys, while the hormone oestrogen in girls stimulates the brain's growth. During growth, the right hemisphere tries to create connections with the left. As the left hemisphere in boys develops more slowly than the right, it appears that more connections within the right hemisphere are created.

Each hemisphere has its own specialisation. Language and linear thinking are located in the left and emotion and physical orientation in the right. Both sides work together through a large, centrally located nerve bundle called the *corpus callosum*. The connection between the two hemispheres is narrower in boys than in girls. The hemispheres need to work together constantly, a prerequisite for reading and speaking about emotions.

In general, boys remain in the gross motor skills phase much longer, which is why it's important that we as parents and educators adjust our activities and our expectations. Indeed, sensorimotor ripening is of the utmost importance. For example, even if a five-year-old boy is cognitively ready for first grade, I would recommend that he not spend his time with cognitive tasks but allow him to spend his energy on tasks that strengthen his sensorimotor foundation first.

In general, girls have a better feeling for language because of the stronger connection between the two hemispheres. Language requires both hemispheres, so it is easier for girls to make connections and perform various tasks at the same time. However, a fast-working brain can cause speed errors. Girls learn by gathering information and by talking about their thoughts, ambitions and emotions.

Boys often focus on a particular subject and learn by becoming completely engrossed in it. They also focus on movement and can work on a physical project endlessly. Their sensorimotor skills are strengthened through continuous repetition. Many boys learn by doing: by trying things out and learning from their mistakes. Boys also need more time to process information, which is why time to rest is so important. Of course, resting time is also crucial for girls, and personal attention remains the most important and valuable development aid parents and educators can give to children, regardless of gender.

Obviously, there's no difference in intelligence between boys and girls. However, our education system is very much based on language, which could give girls an advantage. Additionally, there are developmental differences between girls and boys both socially and emotionally. By taking note of these differences, parents can help their children to fulfil their potential. Parents often ask for advice on how to stimulate the development of their children. The best guidance I can give is to try and discover, whether with a professional or alone, what makes your child enthusiastic, what is difficult for them and how they can best be guided and supported.

Why is play so important in the early years?

Parents and educators want nothing more than to support children in making the most of their talents and abilities. By helping them to develop their abilities, we stimulate them, which is the basis for learning how to 'learn' at school. Basic skills such as hand–eye coordination are needed to write, read and learn maths, and a healthy spirit needs a healthy body. If a child in first grade is tired, listless, has daily headaches or writes illegibly, there's an imbalance that will impede further development of their skills.

During the first seven years of life rapid growth and sensorimotor maturation take up an enormous amount of children's energy. Only around the seventh year, once their adult teeth have started to develop, does this energy become available for cognitive processes. This is the principle on which the Steiner-Waldorf school system is based, and is why exploratory play rather than prescriptive learning should be central in kindergarten.

Why is my nine-year-old so insecure?

I often use the word 'commitment' to explain that children need to learn to be in command of their own body, to feel at home in it. This is a complicated path that we as humans follow right through into adulthood. Once an adult, we still experience moments when we've slept badly and are so tired that we might stumble against a table or miss the last step on the stairs. These moments wake us up and make us move more carefully. In children, this commitment, or learning to be in command of their body, takes place on a number of levels in various phases of their development. These are transitional phases that may be experienced as some kind of 'bump in the road' for children, and can be expressed in behaviour or by becoming physically ill.

Around the tenth year, we see such a bump caused by the physiological change of the child's heart rate gradually slowing down and creating a new physiological balance. This physical change brings a change in experience (soul) in the child. A transition occurs (in Steiner-Waldorf education often referred to as the 'Rubicon'): impressions become coloured by personal feelings. These personal feelings can overwhelm some children – all of a sudden they sleep poorly, overthink minor things or are pre-occupied with how they appear to others. This extreme behaviour is sometimes also called pre-adolescence. If this physiological stage embeds 'insufficiently', children may also experience physical problems (for example, headaches and stomach aches) without specific physical cause.

We could see this transition as the further awakening of the 'I'. It's an enormous change that is often accompanied by insecurity and loneliness. Being in command of their body, having commitment, in this phase is a prerequisite to children being able to stand on their own two feet later in life. As parents, we can support children through this transition by giving them positive personal attention and by setting clear boundaries. Physically, we can support our children by making sure they don't become overly exhausted through too much schoolwork or too many extracurricular activities.

How can I engage my emotional teenager?

Older children in particular often focus intensely on the changes happening in their lives (physically, emotionally and socially). Unfortunately, these changes take up a lot of energy, and children can lose themselves in these periods of transition. Sport, activities or helping around the house encourage them to come into action physically, which in turn engages them on a soul level, which connects with the 'I', sparking interest and enthusiasm. The impasse that occurs through inactivity has far-reaching consequences: during a boring, sedentary class children will slouch in a chair and the subject material will flow over their heads.

Conversely, if your child is physically exhausted through elite sports, lack of sleep or schoolwork, their energy will diminish and they will become tired, lethargic and indifferent. Energy is restored through good nutrition, rest and doing useful outdoor tasks or sports at a less intense level.

12.
Why Don't Children Sit Still?

There is no escaping the fact that children develop and learn through movement. As parents and caregivers our aim shouldn't be to curb or limit this natural tendency in our children, but rather to encourage them to move in the *appropriate* way, according to their age and stage and their individual developmental abilities. Movement means experience, learning and growth, but as a society we often don't use this to its fullest advantage or take into account its importance in the development of the whole human being. Sensorimotor development is more than just the mechanics of bones and muscles – it involves the body's inner processes just as much as its outer actions. Imagine it this way: a child wants to pick an apple from a tree. The apple is the reason why the child stretches out his arm, stands on his tiptoes or climbs up a ladder. The apple becomes the child's incentive to move, unlocking the will and translating his impulse into the movement of picking. The child looks forward to having the apple (soul) and intends (I) to pick it. The apple was already with the child (I) before he started moving. When children take action, they are given the chance to learn using their whole self, through experience and discovery.

As the enabler of experience, movement provides children with stable foundations that will last a lifetime. Ensuring that our children find the best kind of movement for them, to suit their unique, individual development needs, is one of the greatest gifts we can give. Every child will experience stumbling blocks along the way – some seemingly larger than others – but with love, support (both emotional and physical) and encouragement, we can help our children find their way on their own journey of development.

Afterword

Since childhood, being physically active has always been hugely important for me in order to be able to know and experience myself. When I was ten, I had back problems and was given a back brace. After a lot of tears and whining, my parents came to a deal with the orthopaedic surgeon: I was allowed to continue horse riding. This was the best decision they could have made. During the hours spent on the back of a horse, I could get rid of all of my extra energy. It was during this time that I had physiotherapy for my back problems. In hindsight, this period of my youth contributed to my motivation to choose this career, especially working with children. In short, after thirty years, I still feel committed to helping children with their own sensorimotor development and finding their individualism.

All the examples used in this book come from my own practice. The names of the children have been changed. The examples have been summarised and don't do justice to each individual child. This book is absolutely not complete – there are many related subjects and you can find suggested reading listed in the back of this book.

I would very much like to thank all the children and parents I have worked with for their trust. Thank you to all the healthcare professionals with whom I have worked, particularly Joke Butler, friend and paediatrician, for your positive, critical notes. Thank you to Henk, my love, husband and inspiration, for your never-ending attention and support. The paths of our individual goals have intersected frequently over the past thirty years, allowing us to put our energy to various projects in which children are central. 'A child may be a child in order for him to become a complete human being'.

Notes

1. Neural pathways are the connection between nerve cells in the brain. Information processing occurs through continuous adjustments between these connections. Research in neurobiology gives us insight into the workings of the brain.
2. These tips are based on research by the influential paediatrician Dr. Emmi Pikler, whose works are not widely available in English, but who you can read more about online.
3. There is lots of information on the importance of warmth in Edmond Schoorel's *Warmth: Nurturing Children's Health and Wellbeing*, Floris Books, 2017.
4. Research quoted by Manfred Spitzer in *Digitale Demenz* (Digital Dementia: How we Destroy the Minds of Ourselves and Our Children), which is not available in English but which you can read more about online.
5. As above.
6. T. Barabowski et al. in *Huisarts en Wetenschap*, August 2012.
7. Edmond Schoorel explores the impact of digital devices on children's health and education in *Managing Screen Time: Raising Balanced Children in the Digital Age*, Floris Books, 2016.
8. P. van Loon et al., 'Gameboy-generatie verleert gezonde houding' (Problems with posture in the 'Gameboy generation'), in *Medisch Contact*, July 31, 2013.

Further Reading

Aeppli, Willi, *The Care and Development of the Human Senses: Rudolf Steiner's Work on the Significance of the Senses in Education*, Floris Books, UK, 2013.

Bothmer, Fritz von, *Gymnastic Education*, Mercury Press, USA, 2001.

Eijgenraam, Lois, *Helping Children Form Healthy Attachments: Building the Foundation for Strong Lifelong Relationships*, Floris Books, UK, 2017.

Evans, Michael and Iain Rodger, *Healing for Body, Soul and Spirit: An Introduction to Anthroposophic Medicine*, 3rd ed., Floris Books, UK, 2017.

Glöckler, Michaela and Wolfgang Goebel, *A Waldorf Guide to Children's Health*, Floris Books, UK, 2018.

Haren, Wil van and Rudolf Kischnick, *Child's Play 1 & 2: Games for Life for Children and Teenagers*, Hawthorn Press, UK, 1996.

Harvey-Zahra, Lou, *Happy Child, Happy Home: Conscious Parenting and Creative Discipline*, Floris Books, UK, 2014.

Howard, Susan, *The Developing Child: The First Seven Years*, WECAN, USA, 2004.

Jaffke, Freya, *Let's Dance and Sing: Rhythmic Games for the Early Childhood Years*, WECAN, USA, 2017.

—, *Work and Play in Early Childhood*, Floris Books, UK, 1996.

Jantzen, Cornelia, *Dyslexia: Learning Disorder or Creative Gift?*, Floris Books, UK, 2009.

Kiel-Hinrichsen, Monika, *Why Children Don't Listen: A Guide for Parents and Teachers*, Floris Books, UK, 2006.

Kutik, Christiane, *Stress-Free Parenting in 12 Steps*, Floris Books, UK, 2010.

Lievegoed, Bernard, *Phases of Childhood: Growing in Body, Soul and Spirit*, Floris Books, UK, 2005.

Martin, Michael and Wolfgang Schad, *Arts and Crafts in Waldorf Schools*, Floris Books, UK, 2017.

Meijs, Jeanne, *You and Your Teenager: Understanding the Journey*, Floris Books, UK, 2013.

Murray, Lorraine E., *Calm Kids: Help Children Relax with Mindful Activities*, Floris Books, UK, 2012.

Palmer, Sue, *Upstart: The Case for Raising the School Starting Age and Providing What the Under-Sevens Really Need*, Floris Books, UK, 2016.

Schoorel, Edmond, *Managing Screen Time: Raising Balanced Children in the Digital Age*, Floris Books, UK, 2016.

—, *Warmth: Nurturing Children's Health and Wellbeing*, Floris Books, UK, 2017.

Sherborne, Veronica, *Developmental Movement for Children*, 2nd ed., Worth Publishing, UK, 2001.

Siegel, Dr Daniel J. and Dr Tina Payne Bryson, *The Whole-Brain Child: 12 Proven Strategies to Nurture Your Child's Developing Mind*, Little Brown, UK, 2012.

Soesman, Albert, *Our Twelve Senses: How Healthy Senses Refresh the Soul*, Hawthorn Press, UK, 2001.

Spitzer, Manfred, *Digitale Demenz: Wie wir uns und unsere Kinder um den Verstand bringen* (Digital Dementia: How we Destroy the Minds of Ourselves and Our Children), Droemer Verlag, Munich, 2012.

Steiner, Rudolf, *Education for Special Needs: The Curative Education Course (Collected Works of Rudolf Steiner)*, 2nd ed., Rudolf Steiner Press, UK, 2014.

—, *The Foundations of Human Experience*, Anthroposophic Press, USA, 1996.

—, *The Waking of the Human Soul and the Forming of Destiny*, Steiner Book Centre, Canada, 1983.

Tapfer, Barbara and Annette Weisskircher, *An Illustrated Guide to Everyday Eurythmy:, Discover Balance and Self-Healing through Movement*, Floris Books, UK, 2017.

Taylor, Michael, *Finger Strings: A Book of Cat's Cradles and String Figures*, Floris Books, UK, 2008.

Wildgruber, Thomas, *Painting and Drawing in Waldorf Schools: Classes 1 to 8*, Floris Books, UK, 2012.

Resources

WELEDA WEBSITE (UK/USA)

www.weleda.co.uk
www.weleda.com

SHERBORNE DEVELOPMENTAL MOVEMENT WEBSITE (INTERNATIONAL/UK)

www.sherborneinternational.com
www.sherbornemovementuk.org

ROCK AND WATER WEBSITE (UK/USA)
www.rockandwater.org.uk
www.rockandwaterprogram.com

NATURAL TOYS AND WRITING SUPPLIES
www.myriadonline.co.uk

WALDORF SCHOOLS

In 2018 there were over 1,200 Waldorf schools and 2,000 Early Years settings in over 60 countries around the world. Up-to-date information can be found on any of the websites below.

Australia
Association of Rudolf Steiner Schools in Australia
www.steinereducation.edu.au

New Zealand
Federation of Rudolf Steiner Schools
www.rudolfsteinerfederation.org.nz

North America
Association of Waldorf Schools of North America
www.whywaldorfworks.org

South Africa
Southern African Federation of Waldorf Schools
www.waldorf.org.za

UK
Steiner Waldorf Schools Fellowship
www.steinerwaldorf.org.uk

Parenting with Values

12 Essential Qualities Your Children Need and How to Teach Them

Christiane Kutik

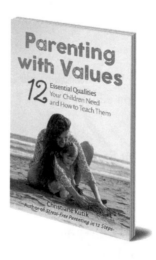

This engaging book encourages parents to reflect on the values they want to pass on to their children. In twelve short, easy-to-digest chapters, Kutik discusses the essential qualities that children need, values like compassion, honesty, respect and self-esteem, and explains how each one is learned and passed on from parent to child.

Filled with everyday examples of values in action, this book will inspire parents who wish to proactively encourage positive development in their children.

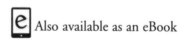 Also available as an eBook

florisbooks.co.uk

Warmth

Nurturing Children's Health and Wellbeing

Edmond Schoorel

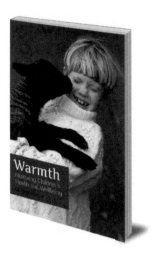

Warmth – this one word has so many powerful, positive associations. As parents we want our children to be warm – physically and emotionally. We raise them to be warm people full of motivation and hope.

In this unique and original book, anthroposophical therapist Edmond Schoorel explores the role of warmth in child development. This practical book offers a valuable insight into raising motivated, healthy children who are self-confident and warm in their relationships.

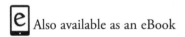 Also available as an eBook

florisbooks.co.uk

Calm Kids

Help Children Relax with Mindful Activities

Lorraine E. Murray

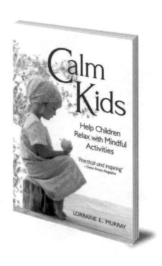

Mindfulness and meditation can help children to recognise and cope with stress and tension. In this useful and inspiring book, Lorraine Murray shows us how to lead fun and peaceful meditation sessions with children.

Suitable for complete beginners or readers already familiar with mindfulness and meditation techniques, Murray suggests ways to help children with hyperactive behaviour or anxiety problems feel calm, happy and relaxed.

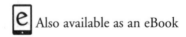 Also available as an eBook

florisbooks.co.uk

Helping Children Form Healthy Attachments

Building the Foundation for Strong Lifelong Relationships

Lois Eijgenraam

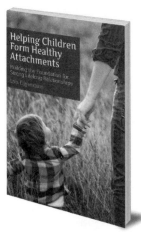

'Practical, easy to read and understand, and very approachable.' – Kindling

Security, trust and self-confidence are all vital for healthy child development. But to build these essential skills, children must rely on healthy bonds with adults and guidance from loving parents and carers. With helpful tips and real case studies, this insightful book will help parents to develop routines, set boundaries and recognise different behavioural patterns.

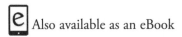 Also available as an eBook

florisbooks.co.uk

Happy Child, Happy Home
Conscious Parenting and Creative Discipline

and

Creative Discipline, Connected Family
Transforming Tears, Tantrums and Troubles While Staying Close to Your Children

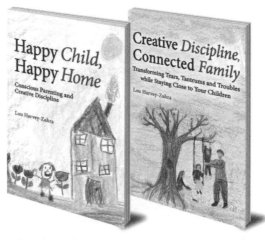

'A practical and inspiring book.' – Juno magazine on Happy Child, Happy Home

In these two inspiring introductions to 'conscious parenting' and managing child behaviour, experienced parenting coach and former Steiner-Waldorf teacher, Lou Harvey-Zahra offers candid advice for parents striving to create a harmonious family home. Packed with case studies and frequently asked questions these books are essential reading material for parents everywhere.

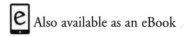 Also available as an eBook

florisbooks.co.uk